Activate More Purpose and Passion in YOU!

90 Day Workbook

Create that AWESOME life you crave!

by Juliana Ericson, Life Counselor Extraordinaire

Dedication

I dedicate this book to all of those who have ever been stuck between a rock and a hard place, not knowing which way to turn or which step to take. I know the feeling.

Introduction

After spending years beating my head against walls making mistake after mistake, I decided to try something completely different. I decided I would learn from people who had experienced adversity and had emerged from their ashes dripping with glory and empowerment. That's when I really began to deepen my spiritual journey. I finally admitted I didn't know how to "do life". Before that, I had merely been dipping my toes in the golden pond of transformation, reading tons of self-help books, attending a plethora of workshops, and talking the talk. I was merely pretending.

I began to live life authentically, admitting when I was wrong and when I was right, seeking out teachers who had experienced what I wanted to learn. I began to fly. I soared above my mistakes, understanding they were merely stepping stones to my greater self. I became the wind, moving effortlessly around obstacles, and over adversity. I learned that nothing could affect me except my beliefs about myself. That was my lesson: I am in charge of my thoughts, no one else.

Activate More Purpose and Passion in YOU!

Create that AWESOME life you crave

LET'S GET STARTED!

I've been a Life Counselor for over 17 years and LOVE IT! My purpose IS my passion. I love helping people live their authentic lives, move through their limitations, live out their dreams and their joys. I intend to help you do that. This workbook will kickstart you in that direction! If you have any questions or comments during the 90 days feel free to post to my blog at www.breathworks.net. Or you may contact me directly.

How this program works......

1: Take a minute to think about what you feel is a basic, long-standing limiting thought you've had your whole life - one that's shown up over and over again for as long as you can remember. It's important that you take the time to really think about what this limiting thought might be. You will be working with this thought's *opposite*, your Love Law, for the next 90 days in this workbook. On the next page I have suggestions to help you uncover the limiting thought **that has held you back for years** from experiencing your fulfilling life.

Along with the new thoughts and actions that are recommended in this workbook, I have some mind-body motions for you to use to cement the new patterns into your body. These might feel odd or even silly at first, but they're a crucial part of the success of this program. You may have read from people like Dr. Deepak Chopra, Louise L. Hay and others that our body has a type of intelligence. It's important to have it aligned with our new thought patterns and this is one way to do that.

2: I want you to get used to loving yourself, if you don't already. Loving yourself is EXTREMELY important for any real success in your life to be possible. I read years ago that we need at least 7 hugs a day, so begin with yourself. I'm asking you to begin each day giving yourself a hug and saying "I love you!". You may resist at first, but hopefully you'll get used to it. :-)

3: Each day you'll have a different thought or action to follow for 30 days. After 30 days repeat them all twice, totaling 90 days of working on your invigorated new thought patterns. The second and third times through will be different from the first because you'll be going deeper and deeper into your subconscious as you get used to loosening up your mind/body.

4: Just before you go to sleep, go over in your head 5 things that went well that day or for things you're grateful for.

Here are some suggestions for you to uncover a basic, limiting thought:

Are there words you say repeatedly in various situations, such as "I can't", "I'm not good enough", "I'm stupid", "I'm not worthy", "Life is too hard", "I'm wrong", "I don't belong", "I'm too afraid". It is very likely that you are telling yourself what your subconscious believes is true. Pick the one phrase that seems to be your main limiting thought. Then write the exact opposite of it. For example, for "I'm not good enough" you would write "I am good enough". For "Life is too hard" write "Life is easy". This opposite statement is your LOVE LAW. You will be using this extremely powerful Love Law every day for the next 90 days to reprogram your brain.

How to do the M-B-C Body Movements:

First, I want to tell you why we're doing these body movements. You can literally rewire your brain by creating NEW neuropathways. In the new science Neurogenesis, or new brain cell development, researchers have found in a number of test subjects that neurons are continuously being formed, even by the elderly! Behavior has a significant affect how many new cells are grown. So now we know you CAN teach an old dog new tricks! Many other studies have shown that changes take place deeper & faster when the mind and body are used in tandem when learning desired changes:

New Behaviors = using mind + body together.

Some behaviors I would like you to use in this book are 3 specific movements <u>as you repeat</u> your new Love Law each morning to yourself. These are the 3 Mind-Body-Connection, or M-B-C, movements:

1. Arms straight out in front of your chest. Clasp your fingers together in front of your chest. Point your thumbs upward. Look at your joined thumbs. Create a large figure 8 with your clasped hands, keeping your thumbs pointed-up, moving to the left & up first. Follow your hands in the figure 8 with only your eyes, don't move your head. As you are doing this movement say out loud your Love Law repeatedly with conviction. Do this for 30 seconds.
2. Put your hands up to your shoulders. Touch your right elbow to your left knee. Then touch your left elbow to your right knee. Do this over and over again repeating your Love Law for 30 seconds.

3. Put both hands on your heart, your right hand under your left hand. Repeat your Love Law for 30 seconds.

Now you're ready to begin your new, Purpose-with-Passion life! It's going to be fun and easy now that you've decided to do this program.

Change is safe!

You've been your old self your whole life; now you're going to be a new self. Let go of what doesn't serve you anymore. You can take some of your previous ways with you if you want to. Let go of whatever parts of your life you want, when you want. You are the designer of your life!

DAY 1:

1. Upon awakening say with enthusiasm "Today I'm open to miracles!"

2. Do M-B-C using your supportive statement, Love Law.

3. Give yourself a hug & say "I love you!"

4. Intend 3 things you will do today that will bring you joy, or simply say "I'm willing to see life differently today." INTEND them, don't just say "I'd like for these to happen". INTENDing them to happen adds more weight to your thoughts, adding expectancy and purpose. Suggestions: call an old friend, say something kind to a stranger, arrive early if you're usually late, leave a "love message" for yourself on your answering machine.

5. Just before sleep go over in your head 5 things that went well today or for which you're grateful.

Notes & Ahas:

DAY 2:

1. Upon awakening say with enthusiasm "Today I'm open to miracles!"

2. Do M-B-C using your supportive statement, Love Law.

3. Give yourself a hug & say "I love you!"

4. Make a point not to be, say or think negatively today. Instead, find something from nature or something else beautiful on which to focus. When you need to redirect your thought to a positive direction, think to yourself "Focus on the beauty. Focus on the beauty."

5. Just before sleep go over in your head 5 things that went well today or for which you're grateful.

Notes & Ahas:

DAY 3:

1. Upon awakening say with enthusiasm "Today I'm open to miracles!"

2. Do M-B-C using your supportive statement, Love Law.

3. Give yourself a hug & say "I love you!"

4. Today notice how often your personal unsupportive thought enters into your mind. How do you react? Do you shrivel inside? Do you get angry with others? Do you "medicate" with food, obsessive behavior, alcohol, cigarettes, shopping? In the moment, lovingly say to yourself your POSITIVE supportive statement. Repeat it as often as you need until you're feeling better.

5. Just before sleep go over in your head 5 things that went well today or for which you're grateful.

Notes & Ahas:

DAY 4:

1. Upon awakening say with enthusiasm "Today I'm open to miracles!"

2. Do M-B-C using your supportive statement, Love Law.

3. Give yourself a hug & say "I love you!"

4. Notice today how much time you waste with mindless emails, excessive TV-watching, complaining. These things drain our bodies' energy. If you want or need to escape, try visualizing your ideal life for one minute. Notice as much sensual details as possible: feel it, smell it, hear it, touch it. This is a mind-ENLIVENING exercise.

5. Just before sleep go over in your head 5 things that went well today or for which you're grateful.

Notes & Ahas:

DAY 5:

1. Upon awakening say with enthusiasm "Today I'm open to miracles!"

2. Do M-B-C using your supportive statement, Love Law.

3. Give yourself a hug & say "I love you!"

4. What was one of your favorite things to do when you were a child? Creating what? Organizing what? Writing what? Making what? Write about what you loved to do from the perspective of yourself as a child.

5. Just before sleep go over in your head 5 things that went well today or for which you're grateful.

Notes & Ahas:

DAY 6:

1. Upon awakening say with enthusiasm "Today I'm open to miracles!"

2. Do M-B-C using your supportive statement, Love Law.

3. Give yourself a hug & say "I love you!"

4. Create a pleasant and orderly place to be your powerful and passionate new self. Clean and organize your office or office space. Make sure you have ample light with a bright lamp. Add a vase of flowers, a scented candle, an empowering poster, a brightly colored pillow on your chair.

5. Just before sleep go over in your head 5 things that went well today or for which you're grateful.

Notes & Ahas:

DAY 7:

1. Upon awakening say with enthusiasm "Today I'm open to miracles!"

2. Do M-B-C using your supportive statement, Love Law.

3. Give yourself a hug & say "I love you!"

4. If you could make one change in the world to make it a better place, what would that be? Any thoughts about how would you begin?

5. Just before sleep go over in your head 5 things that went well today or for which you're grateful.

Note & Ahas:

DAY 8:

1. Upon awakening say with enthusiasm "Today I'm open to miracles!"

2. Do M-B-C using your supportive statement, Love Law.

3. Give yourself a hug & say "I love you!"

4. What's a hobby, joy or activity you did a child that you haven't done since your childhood? Why?

5. Just before sleep go over in your head 5 things that went well today or for which you're grateful.

Notes & Ahas:

DAY 9:

1. Upon awakening say with enthusiasm "Today I'm open to miracles!"

2. Do M-B-C using your supportive statement, Love Law.

3. Give yourself a hug & say "I love you!"

4. Write the names of your 2 favorite friends. List their absolutely FINEST qualities. Call them and tell them these things & how grateful you are for their friendship.

5. Just before sleep go over in your head 5 things that went well today or for which you're grateful.

Notes & Ahas:

DAY 10:

1. Upon awakening say with enthusiasm "Today I'm open to miracles!"

2. Do M-B-C using your supportive statement, Love Law.

3. Give yourself a hug & say "I love you!"

4. Look at the list of your friends' qualities from yesterday. These are qualities you really want in yourself. Write on an index card the top 3 & put the card in your wallet. Look at them often today and breathe them into your heart.

5. Just before sleep go over in your head 5 things that went well today or for which you'r grateful.

Notes & Ahas:

DAY 11:

1. Upon awakening say with enthusiasm "Today I'm open to miracles!"

2. Do M-B-C using your supportive statement, Love Law.

3. Give yourself a hug & say "I love you!"

4. Call an acquaintance you've been wanting to know better. Call him or her inviting to go this week to do the activity you loved to do as a child.

5. Just before sleep go over in your head 5 things that went well today or for which you're grateful.

Notes & Ahas:

DAY 12:

1. Upon awakening say with enthusiasm "Today I'm open to miracles!"

2. Do M-B-C using your supportive statement, Love Law.

3. Give yourself a hug & say "I love you!"

4. Call a shy acquaintance or friend asking to go to a zumba or fun aerobic dance class with you this week (or something else fun & active).

5. Just before sleep go over in your head 5 things that went well today or for which you're grateful.

Notes & Ahas:

DAY 13:

1. Upon awakening say with enthusiasm "Today I'm open to miracles!"

2. Do M-B-C using your supportive statement, Love Law.

3. Give yourself a hug & say "I love you!"

4. Help someone today. Maybe offer a free evening of babysitting to a young family you know, bring dinner to a homebound person, pay for a stranger's dinner in a restaurant, leave a free ice cream cone coupon on a bus bench, thank the woman cleaning your office bathroom with a $10 bill. You get the idea.

5. Just before sleep go over in your head 5 things that went well today or for which you're grateful.

Notes & Ahas:

DAY 14:

1. Upon awakening say with enthusiasm "Today I'm open to miracles!"

2. Do M-B-C using your supportive statement, Love Law.

3. Give yourself a hug & say "I love you!"

4. Give 10% of your paycheck as a tithe to someone who inspires your spirit (whether you know them personally or not). If not 10%, then another substantial amount.

5. Just before sleep go over in your head 5 things that went well today or for which you're grateful.

Notes & Ahas:

DAY 15:

1. Upon awakening say with enthusiasm "Today I'm open to miracles!"

2. Do M-B-C using your supportive statement, Love Law.

3. Give yourself a hug & say "I love you!"

4. Write 25 things you've always wanted to do but haven't......yet.

5. Just before sleep go over in your head 5 things that went well today or for which you're grateful.

Notes & Ahas:

DAY 16:

1. Upon awakening say with enthusiasm "Today I'm open to miracles!"

2. Do M-B-C using your supportive statement, Love Law.

3. Give yourself a hug & say "I love you!"

4. Write your supportive statement twenty times with as much as 20 negative responses you feel within you. This is a very powerful way to flush out your negative subconscious. (You can do this every day for as long as you want)

5. Just before sleep go over in your head 5 things that went well today or for which you're grateful.

Notes & Ahas:

DAY 17:

1. Upon awakening say with enthusiasm "Today I'm open to miracles!"

2. Do M-B-C using your supportive statement, Love Law.

3. Give yourself a hug & say "I love you!"

4. Make a song with your Love Law. Sing the lines to a familiar tune. Sing it often today, preferably out loud.

5. Just before sleep go over in your head 5 things that went well today or for which you're grateful.

Note & Ahas:

DAY 18:

1. Upon awakening say with enthusiasm "Today I'm open to miracles!"

2. Do M-B-C using your supportive statement, Love Law.

3. Give yourself a hug & say "I love you!"

4. Today when someone irritates or hurts your feelings, think of them as a helpless and unhappy young child. not having its needs met. Put your hand on your heart and feel compassion for that child.

5. Just before sleep go over in your head 5 things that went well today or for which you'r grateful.

Notes & Ahas:

DAY 19:

1. Upon awakening say with enthusiasm "Today I'm open to miracles!"

2. Do M-B-C using your supportive statement, Love Law.

3. Give yourself a hug & say "I love you!"

4. List 3 things you've done in your life that you're proud of. Think of these things often today.

5. Just before sleep go over in your head 5 things that went well today or for which you're grateful.

Notes & Ahas:

DAY 20:

1. Upon awakening say with enthusiasm "Today I'm open to miracles!"

2. Do M-B-C using your supportive statement, Love Law.

3. Give yourself a hug & say "I love you!"

4. List 3 people who love you. Think about what they love about you. Write these qualities down for you to see. Think about these qualities during the day.

5. Just before sleep go over in your head 5 things that went well today or for which you're grateful.

Notes & Ahas:

DAY 21:

1. Upon awakening say with enthusiasm "Today I'm open to miracles!"

2. Do M-B-C using your supportive statement, Love Law.

3. Give yourself a hug & say "I love you!"

4. Spend 5 minutes in awe today. Look for something to be amazed at: how a flower grows from a single seed, how a baby grows from a single cell, how does light travel? how does the earth revolve around the sun?

5. Just before sleep go over in your head 5 things that went well today or for which you're grateful.

Notes & Ahas:

DAY 22:

1. Upon awakening say with enthusiasm "Today I'm open to miracles!"

2. Do M-B-C using your supportive statement, Love Law.

3. Give yourself a hug & say "I love you!"

4. Write a love letter to yourself and mail it to yourself.

5. Just before sleep go over in your head 5 things that went well today or for which you'r grateful.

Notes & Ahas:

DAY 23:

1. Upon awakening say with enthusiasm "Today I'm open to miracles!"

2. Do M-B-C using your supportive statement, Love Law.

3. Give yourself a hug & say "I love you!"

4. Today really look into people's eyes today as you communicate. See them as Divine Beings, as you are. Feel love radiating from your heart to theirs.

5. Just before sleep go over in your head 5 things that went well today or for which you're grateful.

Notes & Ahas:

DAY 24:

1. Upon awakening say with enthusiasm "Today I'm open to miracles!"

2. Do M-B-C using your supportive statement, Love Law.

3. Give yourself a hug & say "I love you!"

4. Write 25 more things you've always wanted to do but haven't......yet.

5. Just before sleep go over in your head 5 things that went well today or for which you're grateful.

Notes & Ahas:

DAY 25:

1. Upon awakening say with enthusiasm "Today I'm open to miracles!"

2. Do M-B-C using your supportive statement.

3. Give yourself a hug & say "I love you!"

4. Today, eat only healthy, fresh food today and 8 glasses of water. Think grateful thoughts about your body.

5. Just before sleep go over in your head 5 things that went well today or for which you're grateful.

Notes & Ahas:

DAY 26:

1. Upon awakening say with enthusiasm "Today I'm open to miracles!"

2. Do M-B-C using your supportive statement.

3. Give yourself a hug & say "I love you!"

4. Write down what you imagine your perfect life to look like, feel like, smell like. How do you feel in this perfect life? Remain in this state of feeling your perfect for 5 minutes.

5. Just before sleep go over in your head 5 things that went well today or for which you're grateful.

Notes & Ahas:

DAY 27:

1. Upon awakening say with enthusiasm "Today I'm open to miracles!"

2. Do M-B-C using your supportive statement.

3. Give yourself a hug & say "I love you!"

4. List 5 occupations that are offshoots of your main childhood passion. Which one could you do now? What is one step toward that goal you could do today?

5. Just before sleep go over in your head 5 things that went well today or for which you're grateful.

Notes & Ahas:

DAY 28:

1. Upon awakening say with enthusiasm "Today I'm open to miracles!"

2. Do M-B-C using your supportive statement.

3. Give yourself a hug & say "I love you!"

4. It's important to have help - a team to support your progress. Who do you have in these roles? Find someone. (preferably not all your significant other)

   a.Financial guide _____

   b.Psychological guide _____

   c.Business/success guide _____

   d.Spiritual guide _____

   e.Health guide _____

5. Just before sleep go over in your head 5 things that went well today or for which you're grateful.

Notes & Ahas:

DAY 29:

1. Upon awakening say with enthusiasm "Today I'm open to miracles!"

2. Do M-B-C using your supportive statement.

3. Give yourself a hug & say "I love you!"

4. "Be your best self" also means "looking your best". Ask 3 friends to give you a suggestion on how to improve your appearance. Then do them. Plan a dinner outing to celebrate your new changes!

5. Just before sleep go over in your head 5 things that went well today or for which you're grateful.

Notes & Ahas:

DAY 30:

1. Upon awakening say with enthusiasm "Today I'm open to miracles!"

2. Do M-B-C using your supportive statement.

3. Give yourself a hug & say "I love you!"

4. List 3 things you've been putting off doing that's been holding you back. What's the #1 hardest? Do that one today, preferably in the next hour.

5. Just before sleep go over in your head 5 things that went well today or for which you're grateful.

Notes & Ahas:

Begin day **#1** again twice more, making a total of **90 days**. You will be amazed at how different some of your answers will be the second & third time around!!

YAYYYYY!!!!!!!!!!!!! YOU DID IT!!!

You finished **90 days** of life-enhancing, life-stretching, life-deepening exercises that have moved you in the direction of your passion and purpose.

How do you feel differently from 90 days ago?

It's important to acknowledge your successes, <u>even tiny ones</u>, because they are all steps in the correct direction toward the more purposeful & passionate you! The idea is to feel good:

* Feel good about yourself

* Feel good in your physical body

* Feel good in your emotional body

* Feel good in your spiritual connection

The more you feel good about yourself the more and faster progress you'll make towards your life goals. To be clear, I believe THE BEST life goal is happiness. I'm not just talking about "ha-ha-happiness". I'm talking about authentic, deep happiness which is all about living our purpose and passion.

I am a Holistic Life Counselor. If you'd like more support in creating a life of purpose, and of passion, contact me at www.breathworks.net. I support clients in my office, on Skype and on the phone. I conduct workshops for small to medium groups and for companies.

As an added benefit I use Conscious Breathwork and Forgiveness in my work. I'd love to share with you my powerful holistic approach to a purposeful and passionate life.

Spread the love!

My congratulations gift to you is a free guided visualization of a Purposeful and Passionate life. Go to my website at www.breathworks.net and download the FREE Guided Visualization for Empowered Women. Please feel free to share on my blog about your experiences during the past 90 days. It helps others to hear about what you've learned about yourself - challenges & surprises. Your success is my purpose and joy - I LOVE hearing about them!

I wish you peace, love and passionate unfolding of your true nature,

Juliana

Life Counselor, specializing in Conscious Breathing & Prenatal Psychology

About Juliana

Juliana Ericson has been a Holistic Life Counselor and Therapeutic Breath Teacher for 17 years. She explains how our personal core negative beliefs affect our lives and teaches the power of forgiveness.

Juliana is a specialist in prenatal psychology and compassionately guides clients through gentle processes, such as circular breathing, freeing them from self-defeating thought patterns which might have begun before birth and during the birth process. She is a Loving Relationships Facilitator in Training. She teaches Life Coaching and Breathwork schools, conducts workshops and maintains a private practice in Nashville, Tennessee.

Ericson presents corporate talks about the power of Breathwork, including to Vanderbilt University's Nursing Midwives. Although she is an ordained elder with the Presbyterian Church USA, she is a seeker and uses her passion for the sacred from many other traditions, such as Native American, Sufi, Hindu and Buddhist.

She has also written "The Other F Word: 7 Days to Forgiving Anyone" (Balboa Press), a book to support people moving into freedom from victimhood or blame. Forgiveness means "to let go", but most people have trouble actually doing it. This book has success stories and exact steps on how to forgive anyone in seven days.

For in-person, phone or Skype sessions with Juliana, you may reach her through www.Breathworks.net. Follow her daily inspirational postings on her Facebook page: https://www.facebook.com/Breathetoheal

Juliana is also a professional, award-winning artist and paints in her studio located in Nashville, Tennessee. You can find her work at: www.JulianaNashville.com

www.breathworks.net
www.facebook.com/Breathetoheal
Breathworks on Twitter

www.ingramcontent.com/pod-product-compliance
Lightning Source LLC
Chambersburg PA
CBHW070510290526
45790CB00003B/1177